HERBALISM

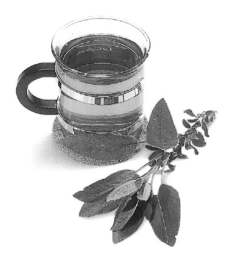

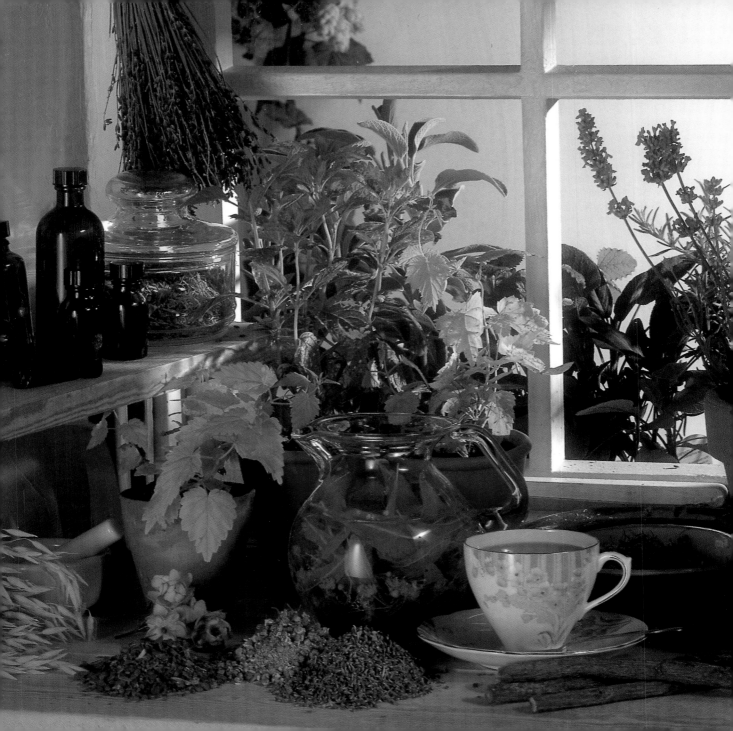

THE NEW LIFE LIBRARY

HERBALISM

USING HERBS FOR STRESS RELIEF

AND COMMON AILMENTS

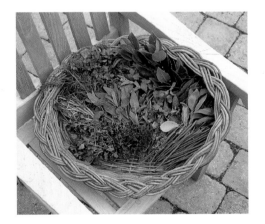

SUE HAWKEY

LORENZ BOOKS

For Cally

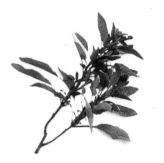
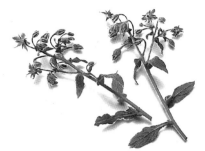

First published by Lorenz Books

© Anness Publishing Limited 1997

Lorenz Books is an imprint of
Anness Publishing Limited
Hermes House
88-89 Blackfriars Road
London SE1 8HA

Published in the USA by Lorenz Books
Anness Publishing Inc., 27 West 20th Street
New York, NY 10011; (800) 354–9657

A CIP catalogue record for this book is available from the British Library

ISBN 1 85967 352 X

Publisher: Joanna Lorenz
Project Editor: Fiona Eaton
Designer: Bobbie Colgate Stone
Photographer: Don Last

Printed in China

5 7 9 10 8 6 4

Publisher's note:
The reader should not regard the recommendations, ideas and techniques expressed and described in this book as substitutes
for the advice of a qualified medical practitioner or other qualified professional. Any use to which the recommendations, ideas
and techniques are put is at the reader's sole discretion and risk.

CONTENTS

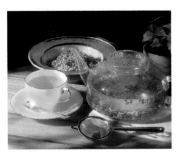

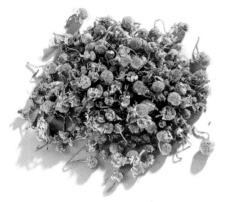

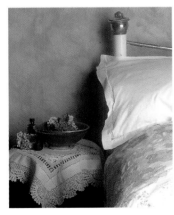

INTRODUCTION

ALL OVER THE WORLD, in all cultures and throughout time, people have used plants not only as food but also for medicinal purposes. Traditional knowledge of herbal remedies used to be passed down from generation to generation, but these days most of us have lost touch with the folklore of herbalism.

In modern industrialized societies, we consume less natural plant material than our ancestors and have a lifestyle that is very different from theirs. At the same time, we have to deal not only with life's normal difficulties and changes, but also with many kinds of pollution, which add in various ways to the stress on our minds and bodies.

Fortunately, the countryside still produces wonderful herbs in abundance, and many can be grown at home. Getting to know the plants growing around you can be a relaxing pleasure in itself. If you learn about their various properties, you can use them to help you feel more healthy and better able to cope with everyday problems. Very simple remedies can be made easily from dried or fresh herbs, and substituting herb tea for stimulating drinks such as tea, coffee and cola will help you to relax and reduce tension.

Herbs, like people, are complex and variable, organic structures made up of many parts. Each plant contains many different constituents combined to give a unique taste and range of actions. Particularly active constituents have been isolated and copied by pharmacists to produce medicines such as aspirin. However, using the whole plant has a more subtle effect and generates fewer side effects. Herbalists therefore prefer to use the whole plant to treat the whole person. Each one of us is unique and reacts to life in a different way. Just as we each have preferences for different foods, we each respond best to particular herbs.

There is much you can do with herbs yourself to treat minor health problems and help your body deal with stress. This book is an introduction to some herbs that can help with stress and other problems, and offers an opportunity to identify some herbal remedies that may be useful to you. Don't forget, though, that trained medical herbalists have a specialized knowledge of plant remedies and medicine. Any problem that fails to respond to the remedies suggested here should be taken to a qualified practitioner.

STRESS AND THE NERVOUS SYSTEM

The involuntary or autonomic nervous system has two divisions. The sympathetic part prepares you for action and initiates the "fight-or-flight" response. The parasympathetic system is responsible for the body's "housekeeping," ensuring good digestion, assimilation of nutrients, detoxification and elimination of waste products. The sympathetic system allows you to respond to stimulation – making the heart and lungs more active

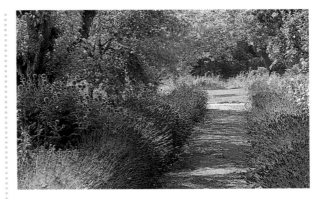

Simply walking down a path of richly scented lavender can help to raise the spirits.

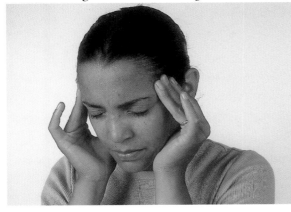

Lavender oil rubbed into the temples encourages relaxation and can help relieve headaches.

and suppressing processes such as digestion and elimination. All life follows a natural rhythm, with periods of activity followed by periods of rest. This is as it should be. Too much stimulation, or an overreaction to stimulation, leads to a state of stress.

If you are subjected to excess stimulation, sympathetic activities become dominant or habitual and may cause you to reach a state of exhaustion, reducing your ability to react and cope appropriately with new stress. This can cause forgetfulness, panic, exhaustion or increased vulnerability to infection. At the same time, reduced parasympathetic activity can cause all sorts of digestive and nutritional debilities as well as poor elimination, which in turn can result in problems with the skin, muscles or joints.

HERBS AND THE NERVOUS SYSTEM

It is our nervous system that coordinates all the complex activities that keep us well and help us adjust to constantly changing circumstances. This book describes some of the beautiful plants that, among their many properties, can be used to support the nervous system. Herbalists call such plants nervines.

NERVOUS TONICS

These plants aid recovery from stress and are useful when we feel debilitated and exhausted after illness, prolonged pressure or trauma. They improve the health and functioning of nervous tissue by invigorating and restoring it.

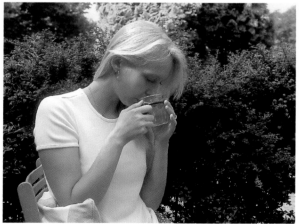

Drinking herb teas is a gentle and simple way to soothe both body and mind.

Some act as gentle stimulants while others are slightly sedating. Your choice will depend on whether nervous debility makes you hyperactive (choose relaxing nervines) or restless, depressed and tired (choose stimulating nervines).

STIMULATING TONICS:
- Wild oats (*Avena sativa*)
- St. John's wort (*Hypericum perforatum*)
- Damiana (*Turnera diffusa*)
- Sage (*Salvia officinalis*)
- Mugwort (*Artemisia vulgaris*)

RELAXING TONICS:
- Skullcap (*Scutellaria lateriflora*)
- Vervain (*Verbena officinalis*)
- Wood betony (*Stachys betonica*)

STIMULANTS

Some plants, such as coffee and tea, stimulate our nervous system without nourishing it. Such over-stimulation is exhausting and so additional herbal stimulants are rarely used. There is a place for gently stimulating nervines, however. For example, mugwort is beneficial during convalescence and rosemary, by stimulating blood flow to the head, is useful in treating tension headaches.
- Rosemary (*Rosmarinus officinalis*)

RELAXANTS AND SEDATIVES

You can use relaxing nervines to calm yourself down and prevent over-stimulation. These relaxing herbs will encourage rest and sleep.

- Lime blossom (*Tilia x europaea*)
- Lavender (*Lavandula spp.*)
- Lemon balm (*Melissa officinalis*)
- Marjoram (*Origanum vulgare*)
- Chamomile (*Chamaemelum nobile* and *Chamomilla recutita*)
- Cramp bark (*Viburnum opulus*)
- Valerian (*Valeriana officinalis*)
- Motherwort (*Leonurus cardiaca*)
- Peppermint (*Mentha piperita*)
- Lady's mantle (*Alchemilla xanthochlora*)
- Californian poppy (*Eschscholzia californica*)
- Hops (*Humulus lupulus*)
- Passionflower (*Passiflora incarnata*)
- Pasque flower (*Anemone pulsatilla*)

ADAPTOGENS

- Korean ginseng (*Panax spp.*)
- Siberian ginseng (*Eleutheroccocus senticosus*)

OTHER USEFUL HERBS

- Licorice (*Glycyrrhiza glabra*)
- Borage (*Borage officinalis*)
- Chaste tree (*Vitex agnus-castus*)
- Evening primrose (*Oenothera biennis*)

CHOOSING REMEDIES

Like all herbs, nervines have a range of actions – choose the one that fits your own symptoms of stress and to which you feel drawn. Knowing, growing, harvesting and drying herbs will improve your relationship with them, and you will find them more helpful.

You may discover that a particularly troubling symptom can be treated by several different remedies. Studying the whole range of symptoms that each herb is known to help can lead you to find one that will help other seemingly unconnected problems. This will be a particularly effective remedy for you.

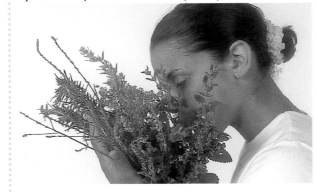

The smell of herbs is very powerful, and they can affect emotions at a very deep level.

PREPARING HERBS

IF YOU GROW herbs in your garden they can be used fresh (except pasque flower), or harvested when they are abundant and dried for future use. Simple herbal remedies can be made up for use either internally or externally. Many herbs are, of course, a delicious addition to food, or they can be taken internally in a variety of other forms: as teas, decoctions, tinctures, inhalations, capsules and powders.

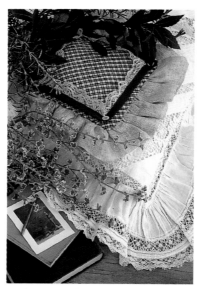

Relaxing herbs such as hops and lavender can be combined in a sleep pillow.

Externally, herbs can be applied as compresses, poultices, ointments, creams or infused oils. You can also add fresh herbs or herbal oils to your bath for a therapeutic soak.

Essential oils, fluid extracts and tablets are usually produced industrially and are not suitable for making at home.

Facing page: Simple herbal remedies can be made easily and cheaply using everyday kitchen equipment.

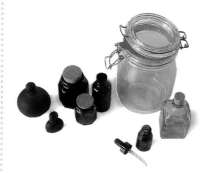

Herbal preparations need to be stored in airtight containers. Dark glass is best for long-term storage of tinctures and oils.

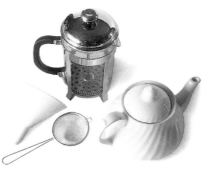

Teas from fresh and dried herbs can be made in a teapot or cafetière.

CAUTION
• Avoid all strong herbal teas during the first three months of pregnancy.
• Do not give peppermint or sage tea to children under four years of age.
• Avoid ready-made herbal mixes that contain sugar.

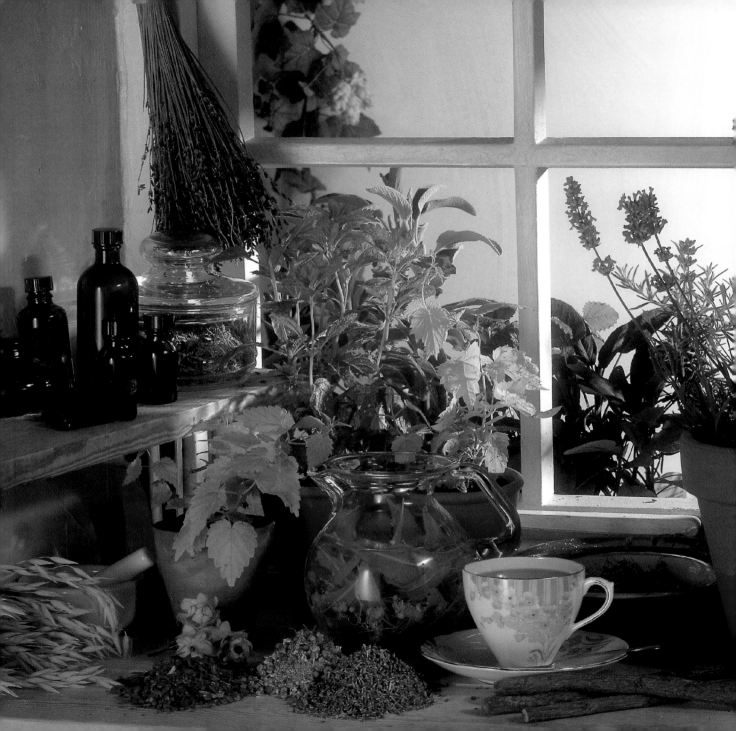

GATHERING AND STORING HERBS

Identifying, growing and harvesting herbs can be a healing experience in itself. Handling herbs will bring you closer to nature and increase your appreciation of the amazing vitality of plants.

GROWING

The best way to acquire herbs to help keep you well is, of course, to grow them yourself. This way you can be sure of what they are and that they are healthy, organically grown and fresh. Most of the herbs used in the remedies in this book will grow well in temperate climates. Many are usually considered to be weeds and actually thrive on disturbed ground and with little care. They bring a sense of vitality to a garden, and being among them and harvesting them is enlivening.

GATHERING

The aerial parts of herbs (the flowers, stems and leaves) should be gathered for use or for drying when the plants are in bud and totally dry. Roots should be dug in the autumn, cleaned and chopped into small pieces.

If you harvest from the wild, make quite sure that you have identified the plant correctly (use a good wildflower book) and that it is not polluted by fertilizers, pesticides or car emissions. Never pick so much that you reduce next year's growth.

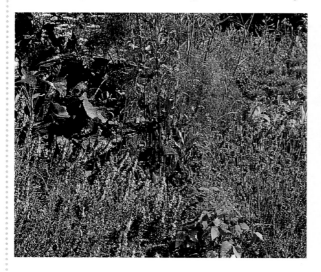

Many of the herbs found in gardens today have been used by herbalists for over two thousand years.

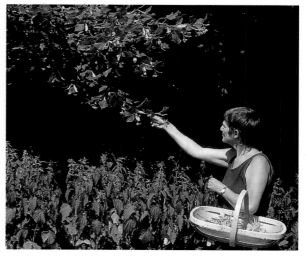

Lime blossom is abundant for easy picking in both the countryside and urban areas during early summer.

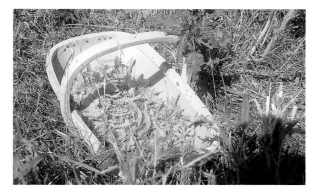

Freshly picked lime blossom ready for drying or for using fresh to make a tea or tincture.

DRYING

Spread your herbs out to dry naturally in an airy position out of direct sunlight. The surroundings should be very dry. Small quantities can be dried effectively in loosely sealed paper bags.

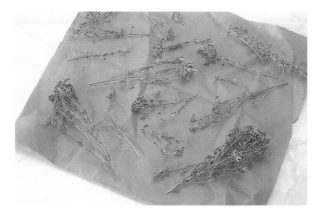

St. John's wort dries well. Spread the stems out evenly to dry and prevent them from touching each other.

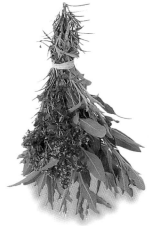

Herbs dry well when hanging in a dry, airy place, out of direct sunlight.

STORING

Store dried herbs in separate, airtight containers away from the light. Don't forget to label and date them. They will keep for up to six months.

Instead of drying your herbs, you can store them in the freezer. This is especially useful for herbs such as lemon balm and parsley, which lose their flavor when they are dried.

BUYING

Many stores stock dried herbs. Buy these only if they seem fresh – they should be brightly colored and strongly aromatic.

Some herbal remedies are now readily available over the counter in the form of capsules, tablets or tinctures. These are usually of good quality. Choose the simpler ones that tell you exactly the type and quantity of herb involved.

13

MAKING TEAS

Herbal teas are also called infusions or tisanes, and are a simple and delicious way of extracting the goodness and flavor from the aerial parts of herbs. You can use either fresh or dried herbs to make a tea (use twice as much fresh plant material as dried). If you find the taste of some herb teas bitter, they can be sweetened with a little honey or flavored by stirring with a licorice stick or adding slices of fresh ginger.

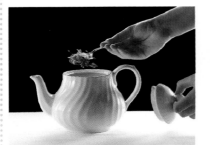

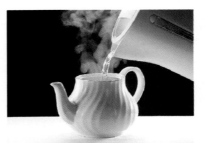

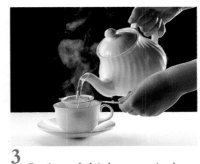

1 Put your chosen herb or herbs into a pot or cup. A standard-strength tea is made with 1 tea-spoon dried or 2 teaspoons fresh herb to each cup of water.

2 Add boiling water, cover with a lid and let steep for 10 – 15 minutes.

3 Strain and drink as required. Teas can be drunk hot or cold. They can be re-heated.

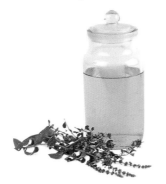

Left: Teas will keep in the fridge in a covered container for up to 24 hours.
Right: Herb teas can also be made in a cafetière. Simply fill the cafetière with the fresh or dried herbs and add boiling water. Allow to steep for 10-15 minutes before pressing down the plunger.

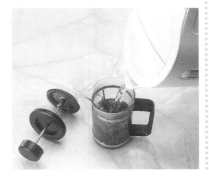

MAKING DECOCTIONS

Infusing in boiling water is not enough to extract the constituents from roots or bark. This harder plant material needs to be boiled, and the resulting liquid is called a decoction. Use a stainless steel, glass or enameled pan, not aluminum, to prepare decoctions.

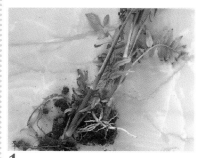

1 Roots and barks need to be harvested in the autumn and prepared for use.

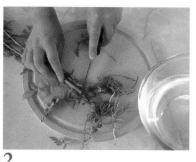

2 Trim the aerial parts of the plant away from the root.

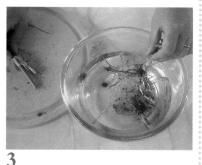

3 Wash the roots thoroughly in clean water, then chop them into small pieces.

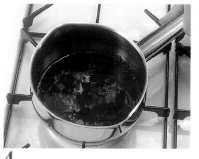

4 Fill a pan with cold water and add 1 teaspoon of the chopped herb material per cup of water. Bring to a boil and simmer for 10 – 15 minutes.

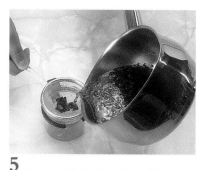

5 Strain off the liquid and let cool before drinking. Decoctions, like teas, can be kept for 24 hours in the fridge. They can be drunk hot or cold.

NERVINES SUITABLE FOR DECOCTIONS
- Valerian
- Licorice
- Cramp bark

Avoid licorice if you have high blood pressure.

MAKING TINCTURES

Sometimes it is more convenient to take a spoonful of medicine rather than make a tea or decoction. Tinctures are made by steeping herbs in a mixture of alcohol and water. The alcohol extracts the medicinal constituents and also acts as a preservative.

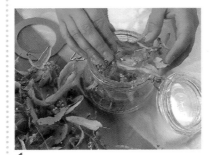

1 Place 4 ounces dried herbs or 11 ounces fresh herbs in a jar.

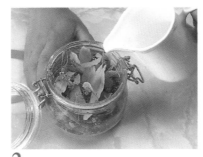

2 Add 1 cup vodka and 1 cup water.

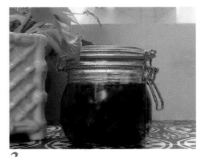

3 Let the herbs steep in the liquid for a month, preferably on a sunny windowsill. Gently shake the jar daily.

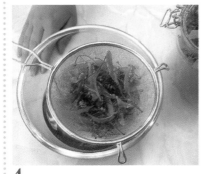

4 Strain and store the tincture in a dark glass bottle (it will keep up to 18 months).

MAKING SYRUPS

Herb syrups make good remedies for giving to children. They also improve the flavor of bitter herbs such as motherwort and vervain.

1 Place 1¼ pounds sugar or honey in a pan and add 4 cups water.
2 Heat gently, stirring, to dissolve the sugar or honey.
3 Add 5 ounces plant material and heat gently for 5 minutes.
4 Turn off the heat and let steep overnight.
5 Strain and store in an airtight container for future use. The sugar acts as a preservative, so a herb syrup will keep for 18 months.

COLD INFUSED OILS

Herbal oils are suitable for external use in massage, as bath oils or for conditioning the hair and skin. Cold infused oils are simple to prepare and are an effective way to infuse delicate flowerheads such as St. John's wort and chamomile.

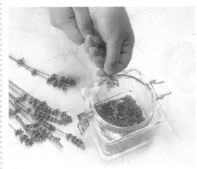

1 Fill a glass storage jar with the flowers or leaves of your chosen dried herb.

2 Pour in a light vegetable oil to cover the herbs – try sunflower or grape seed oil.

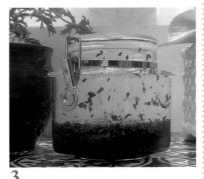

3 Let the jar stand on a sunny windowsill for a month to steep. Give it a shake every day.

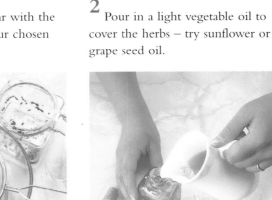

4 Strain the flowers or leaves. For a stronger infusion, renew the herbs in the oil every two weeks.

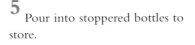

5 Pour into stoppered bottles to store.

USEFUL HERBS FOR MAKING INFUSED OILS
- Rosemary
- Lavender
- St. John's wort
- Chamomile
- Marjoram

Do not put St. John's wort oil on the skin before going into bright sunshine.

HERBS AND FOOD

Plants are very nutritious. They are our main source of vitamins and minerals and provide carbohydrates, protein and roughage. The plants usually called herbs are particularly potent. This points out the narrow divide between food and medicine – a well-nourished body is less likely to get ill. Nettle, for example, contains iron and vitamin C. Kelp contains sodium, potassium, calcium, magnesium, iron, zinc, copper, aluminum and silica as well as vitamin B1 (thiamin). Alfalfa also makes a good multivitamin and mineral supplement since it contains all the vitamins as well as calcium, magnesium, phosphorus and potassium.

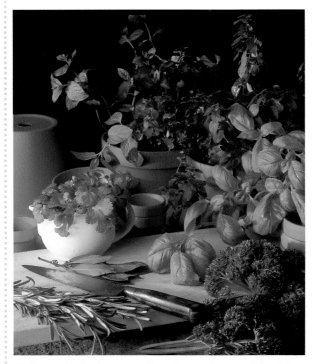

Culinary herbs improve digestion and general health as well as taste delicious.

Knowing about the nutritional value of herbs can change your attitude toward cooking. Adding generous portions of herbs to food becomes more than just adding flavor. Herbs can also be added fresh to salads as a pleasurable way of avoiding nutritional deficiencies.

The wild plants from which some cultivated vegetables were developed are still useful to herbalists. Wild carrot *(Daucus carota)* is a common plant used for urinary problems and to improve digestion. Wild lettuce *(Lactuca virosa)* is a mild sedative and painkiller used to reduce irritable coughs and restlessness.

Not only is what you eat important, but the efficiency with which food is absorbed is crucial. Many herbs stimulate digestive enzymes and encourage efficient intestinal activity. Some of these are still used as culinary herbs: Fennel, caraway, dill and cumin all contain antispasmodic oils which reduce colic. Bitter herbs such as dandelion encourage liver function. Others, such as senna, encourage bowel activity.

Experiment with herbs in food. *A Modern Herbal* by Maud Grieve (1931) is a fascinating source of information and contains many old recipes.

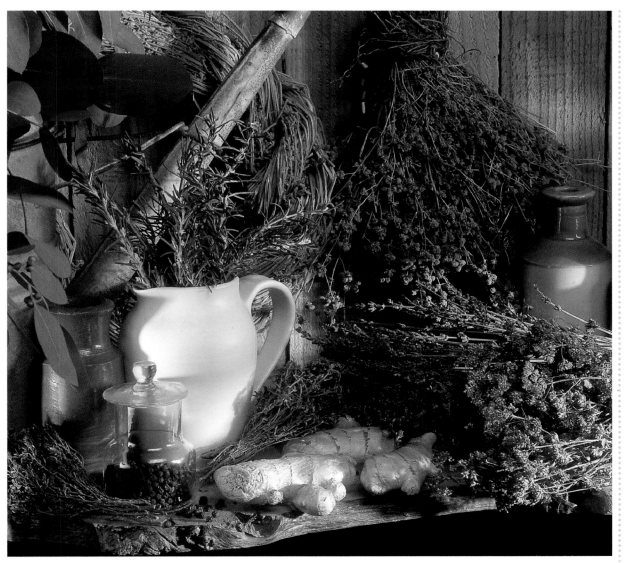

Many of the culinary herbs we use today were distributed throughout Europe by the Roman army.

GUIDE TO HERBS AND THEIR USES

THE HERBS DESCRIBED on the following pages are particularly useful for managing stress and other common conditions. Reading about them and studying the pictures will help you to decide which would be most beneficial for you. You may want to try several before deciding which you find most helpful. Herbs do not usually work instantly, so give them at least two weeks to begin to take effect. If you do not feel better in three weeks, seek the help of a qualified practitioner. Herbs can be used in various combinations, and you will find suggestions for combining them to provide additional benefits.

Most of us would benefit from a nerve tonic during stressful times of our lives. Select an herbal remedy that best suits your symptoms. For example, if when under stress you start to feel depressed, you should look for a stimulating herbal tonic such as wild oats. If, however, stress makes you anxious with symptoms such as palpitations, sweating and sleeplessness, turn toward relaxing herbs.

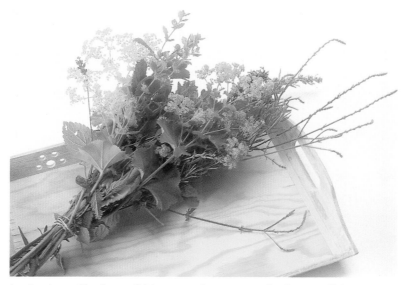

A selection of herbs useful in managing stress and other conditions.

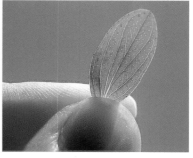

Above: Correct identification is very important. *Hypericum perforatum* is the only St. John's wort with oil glands in the leaves. The glands look like tiny holes when held towards the light. Facing page: Lavender is grown in Europe for its essential oils.

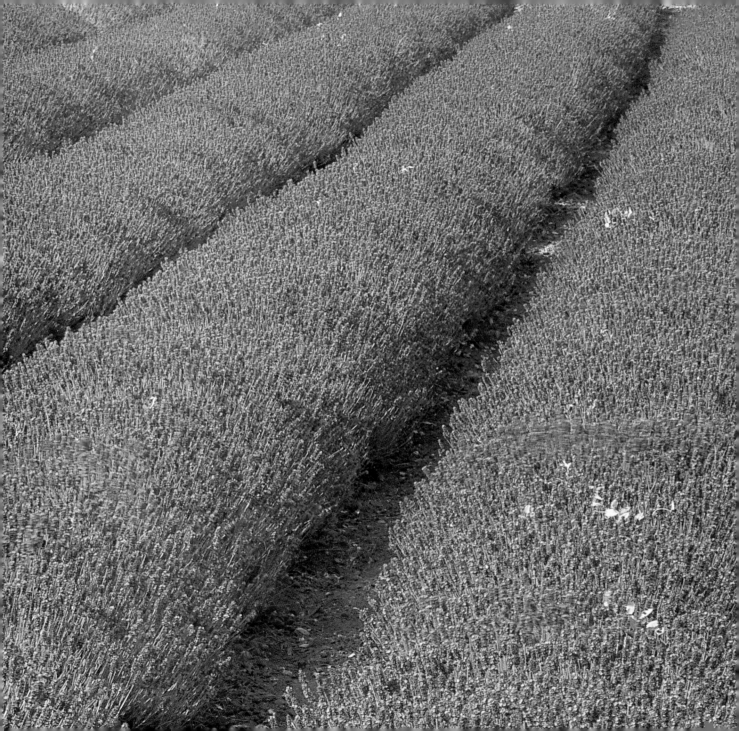

CHAMOMILE

GERMAN CHAMOMILE *CHAMOMILLA RECUTITA* OR ROMAN CHAMOMILE *CHAMAEMELUM NOBILE*

This pretty little daisy is one of the better known herbs, possibly because it is so useful. Its nature is friendly and supportive, both to people and to other plants. It has been called "the plants' physician" because other species growing near it seem to thrive. Use the flowerheads alone in a tea or tincture to relax both the digestive function and those gut feelings that may sometimes disturb you. It makes a very suitable tea to drink late in the day, as it has the opposite effect of coffee, which exacerbates tension and anxiety.

Known as "mother of the gut," chamomile reduces spasms and inflammation in the digestive system as it improves liver function with its bitter action. This makes it an ideal after-dinner drink, especially as it also promotes relaxation. Many people swear by chamomile tea as the ideal bedtime

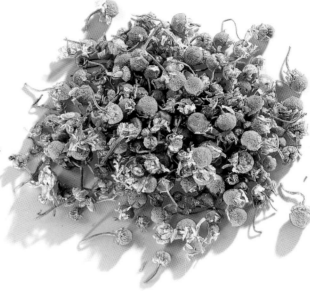

Dried chamomile flowers.

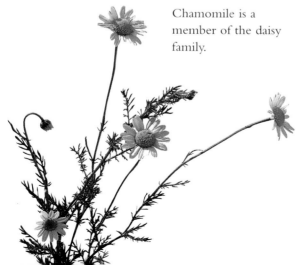

Chamomile is a member of the daisy family.

drink. This gentle plant can also be used to soothe restless babies and children.

Tea bags are convenient but an infusion of loose flowers usually makes a quality tea. Be sure that those you buy are fresh: they should be recognizable flower-heads, bright yellow and white. Inhaling the steam from a cup of chamomile tea reduces the effects of nasal irritants and soothes symptoms of hay fever or rhinitis. Tea bags can also be added to the bath for relaxation.

PARTS USED: Flowerheads.

DOSE: 1 teaspoon dried/2 teaspoons fresh to a cup of boiling water.

LEMON BALM

MELISSA OFFICINALIS, BEE BALM

This plant has so much vitality that it can spread all over the garden. Also called bee balm, it is so much enjoyed by bees that it has been suggested that hives rubbed with the plant will keep the bees close and encourage others to join the hives.

With its lemon-honey scent and tiny white flowers, lemon balm makes a suitable drink for every day, hot in the winter and iced in the summer. This is one of the few herbs which doesn't keep its flavor when dry, so if you have a garden you would be well advised to pick it fresh daily – a constructive way to restrain its rampant habit! If you want to use it in the winter, the best solution is to freeze it. Pick it in early summer when abundant, and freeze it in a plastic container.

Lemon balm supports digestion and relaxation, and is helpful for sensitive digestive systems. It is much used for irritable bowels, nervous indigestion, anxiety and depression. Drinking lemon balm tea also encourages a clear head, so it is useful when you are studying. It makes a good bedtime drink, promoting peaceful sleep and relaxation.

Lemon balm combines well with chamomile.

PARTS USED: Leaves and flowers.

DOSE: 1 teaspoon to a cup of boiling water, up to 4 times a day.

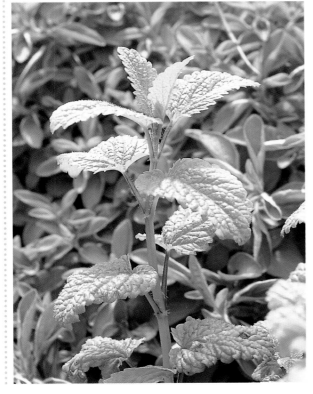

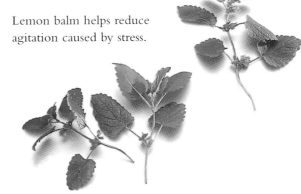

Lemon balm helps reduce agitation caused by stress.

WOOD BETONY

STACHYS BETONICA syn. *S. OFFICINALIS, BETONICA OFFICINALIS*, BISHOP'S WEED
An attractive plant with purple flowers growing out of a satisfying cushion of leaves, wood betony restores the nervous system, especially if headaches and poor memory are a problem. It has the effect of encouraging blood flow to the head.

It has always been a very popular remedy throughout Europe and is also called bishop's weed, perhaps because it was often planted on holy ground. A wide range of beneficial qualities have been ascribed to wood betony and it is certainly worth trying if you are troubled by headaches or migraines.

PARTS USED: Aerial parts.
DOSE: 1 teaspoon dried/2 teaspoons fresh herb to a cup of boiling water.

CAUTION
Avoid high doses during pregnancy.

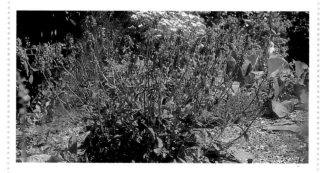

The flowers of wood betony appear in midsummer.

SKULLCAP

SCUTELLARIA LATERIFLORA
This herb is another nervous tonic. It was traditionally associated with the head, because it produces skull-like seed pods. It is very calming, having the same effect as a gentle hand placed on the head. Skullcap can help the anxiety and restlessness that often accompany an overload of worries or responsibilities. Its bitter taste encourages the liver to remove toxins from the body; this includes excess hormones that are often responsible for premenstrual tension.

PARTS USED: Aerial parts, harvested after flowering.
DOSE: 1 teaspoon dried/2 teaspoons fresh herb to a cup of boiling water.

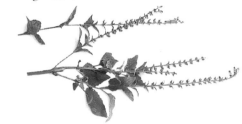

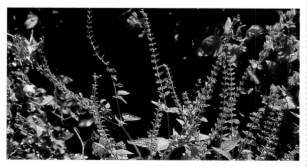

Skullcap takes its name from the skull-like seed pods.

GINSENG

KOREAN GINSENG, *PANAX SPP.*

The name of this plant means "wonder of the world." By improving the production of adrenal hormones, Korean ginseng helps the body to adapt to stress and resist disease. Because it is stimulating, prolonged use could be exhausting, but as a short-term remedy for fatigue or debility, it is very effective.

In China, small doses are taken to support health in the elderly and to protect from serious disease. Korean ginseng also has a reputation as an aphrodisiac and induces energy of every type. In the west it is usually prescribed during periods of particular stress or to those suffering from debilitating diseases.

SIBERIAN GINSENG, *ELEUTHEROCOCCUS SENTICOSUS*

Siberian ginseng is a European plant which, like Korean ginseng, improves the ability to adapt to stress. It is less stimulating, but increases stamina and skilled performance.

Both Korean and Siberian ginseng improve clarity of mind and are helpful when preparing for exams or other demanding projects.

PARTS USED: Dried root.

DOSE: 1 gram per day or as instructed for shorter periods.

CAUTION
- Avoid the use of ginseng during pregnancy or with other stimulants.
- Do not take high doses for more than six weeks without expert advice.
- Stop taking ginseng if it makes you feel agitated or you develop a headache.

Ginseng is a common over-the-counter remedy. Make sure it is of good quality – usually the more expensive brands are better.

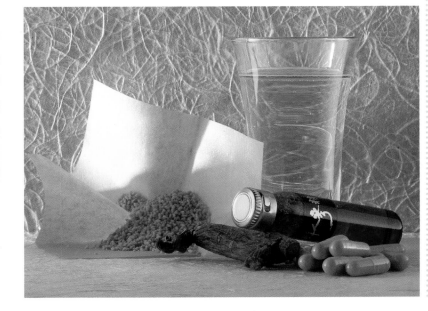

LICORICE

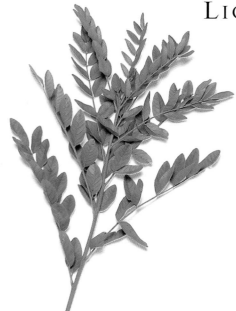

Licorice is a member of the pea family.

GLYCYRRHIZA GLABRA

This is an extremely useful herb which has been cultivated since the Middle Ages for its sweet, aromatic roots. Among its many actions is its beneficial effect on digestion; it reduces inflammation all along the gut and encourages bowel activity – licorice is the basis of most proprietary laxatives. It is often used as a flavoring and will not raise blood sugar levels. If you like it, add a little to sweeten any herb tea – just stand a stick in the cup until you achieve the desired sweetness. Under close supervision, the root can be given to babies to chew and will ease the pain of teething.

Licorice also supports the adrenal glands and is therefore useful in any inflammatory condition such as eczema or arthritis. It will help to restore natural steroid production after a course of steroid medication. Since stress requires the adrenal glands to keep producing adrenaline, it may be that people who love to eat licorice daily are instinctively seeking support for stressful times or lifestyles.

Licorice heated in honey makes a soothing syrup that helps to relax the chest in conditions such as bronchitis and asthma.

PARTS USED: The root (licorice sticks) or solidified juice in the form of black bars.

DOSE: 1 teaspoon to a cup of boiling water.

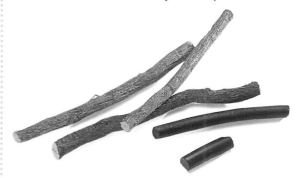

Licorice sticks are sections of root. The black bars are made of solidified juice and are very strong.

CAUTION
Licorice is not recommended for those with high blood pressure.

BORAGE

BORAGO OFFICINALIS

This strapping plant, with bristly and fleshy stems and leaves, sports surprisingly exotic, luminous blue flowers. These are traditionally used in drinks to raise the spirits. They make an attractive garnish to many dishes, especially ice cream and other cold summer desserts. Traditionally associated with courage, borage improves the production of adrenaline and is therefore, like licorice, useful during stressful times or after steroid medication.

This plant is very nutritious, containing calcium, potassium and traces of gamma linoleic acid. It also helps in the absorption of iron. Oil from the seeds is a good alternative to evening primrose oil in treating skin disease or rheumatism. It is commercially available in capsules and is sometimes called Starflower oil.

In addition to bringing "courage and good heart," borage increases milk production in nursing mothers and is a useful herb to take during fevers, infections and convalescence.

PARTS USED: Leaves, flowers and seeds. The leaves, being so fleshy, need to be dried quickly and are best heated very gently in a cool oven until crisp.

DOSE: 1 teaspoon dried/2 teaspoons fresh to a cup of boiling water.

"Borage cheers the heart and raises drooping spirits."
DIOSCORIDES

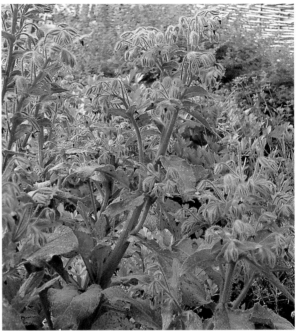

Borage is a rampant plant and seeds itself easily.

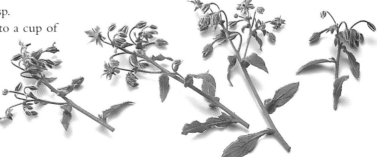

HOPS

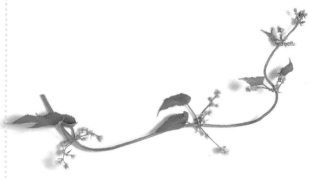

The twining stem of the fast-growing hop vine.

HUMULUS LUPULUS

The name hop comes from the Anglo-Saxon *hoppen*, "to climb"—the twining fibrous stems may reach some 15 feet in height. Like hemp, fiber from the stems was at one time used to make coarse fabric and paper. Nowadays the plant is best-known for its use in brewing; beer made with hops replaced traditional herb ales made from malt and cleared with ground ivy. Hops have the advantage of flavoring as well as clearing beer, but their introduction remained controversial for many years and Henry VIII forbade their use, as they "spoiled the taste and endangered the people." Hops were thought to provoke melancholy, and their use is still not advised for those who are feeling depressed. Hops are also known to reduce sexual potency.

Hops are taken as a bitter tonic which improves digestion and reduces restlessness. It also has a sedative effect and will provoke deep sleep. The action is due, in part, to the presence of volatile oils, which give the characteristic odor and make pillows stuffed with dried hops useful for restless sleepers.

The tender young shoots can be eaten raw or cooked and eaten like asparagus in the spring.

PARTS USED: Dried flowers from the female plant, called "strobiles."

DOSE: Not more than 1 teaspoon a day.

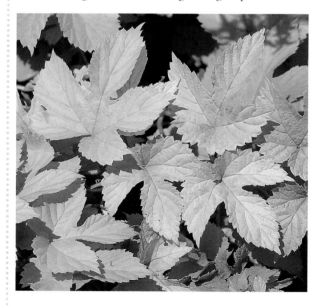

Golden hops are so called because of their brightly colored leaves.

CAUTION
Avoid the use of hops when depressed.

VALERIAN

VALERIANA OFFICINALIS, ALL HEAL

This Valerian is not the jolly red or white plant seen decorating walls (*Centranthus ruber*), but a tall herb with whitish-pink flowers that grows in damp places. When dried, the root has a characteristic earthy smell that attracts cats.

Valerian root has a powerful sedative effect on the nervous system and reduces tension and anxiety very effectively. It can be used to reduce hyperactivity, palpitations, spasm, period pain and tranquilizer withdrawal. It is especially useful if anxiety makes sleep difficult.

PARTS USED: Dried root.

DOSE: 1 teaspoon to a cup of boiling water at bedtime.

CAUTION
High doses taken over a long period may cause headaches.

Valerian roots are harvested after the leaves have died.

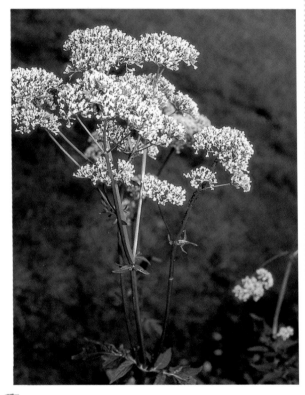

Valerian grows in damp woods and meadows.

PASSIONFLOWER

PASSIFLORA INCARNATA, MAYPOP

This is a climbing plant that produces spectacular flowers and edible fruit. The species used medicinally prefers a warm, sunny climate. Buy it dried from a supplier to make sure you get the right plant.

Passionflower is often included in sleeping mixes and is very helpful for restlessness and insomnia. It seems to counteract the effects of adrenaline, thus reducing the "fight-or-flight" response that may cause anxiety, palpitations or nervous tremors.

It is also used as a painkiller to ease neuralgia and the pain of shingles.

PARTS USED: Dried leaves and flowers.

DOSE: ¼ – ½ teaspoon dried herb twice a day, or 1 teaspoon at night, or take an over-the-counter preparation as directed.

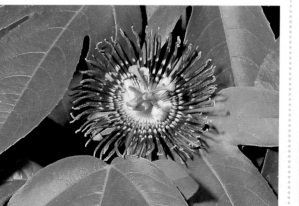

Passionflower is said to resemble Christ's thorn crown.

CALIFORNIAN POPPY

ESCHSCHOLZIA CALIFORNICA

The beautiful, delicate flowers last for only one day, then disappear to be replaced by long, pointed seed pods. The stunning hot orange, yellow and pinkish colors of the blooms perhaps account for its French name, *globe de soleil*.

Californian poppy is a gentle painkiller and sedative that reduces spasm and over-excitability. It combines well with passionflower.

PARTS USED: The whole plant, dried.

DOSE: 1 teaspoon dried herb to a cup of boiling water.

CAUTION
Avoid this herb if you suffer from glaucoma.

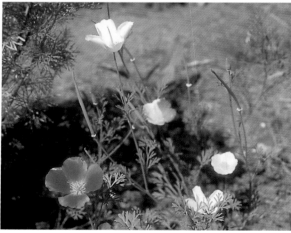

The Californian poppy thrives in sun and poor soil.

SAGE

SALVIA OFFICINALIS

A beautiful, evergreen plant with fine purple flowers in early summer, sage looks strong and supportive. Like many culinary herbs, it aids digestion, while the familiar aroma recalls roast dinners.

It has antiseptic properties and can be used as a compress on wounds that are slow to heal, or as a gargle or mouthwash for infections of the mouth or throat. It is also said that it will darken graying hair if used as a rinse.

Sage reduces secretions; it can be used to slow milk production during weaning and to reduce night sweats and menopausal hot flashes. During menopause its beneficial action is supported by the slight estrogen content of the herb.

For the nervous system, Culpeper described sage as warming, improving the memory and quickening the senses. It is recommended for debility and confusion and has been associated with longevity.

PARTS USED: Leaves and flowers.

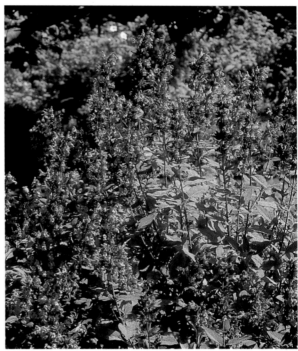

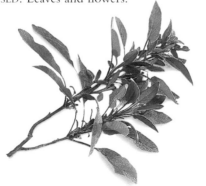

Sage is currently being investigated as a possible remedy for Alzheimer's disease.

DOSE: 1 teaspoon dried/2 teaspoons fresh to a cup of boiling water.
If taking sage regularly at therapeutic doses, take for three weeks, then miss a week before continuing.

CAUTION
Avoid during pregnancy.

Sage can be toxic at high doses or over long periods.

31

MUGWORT

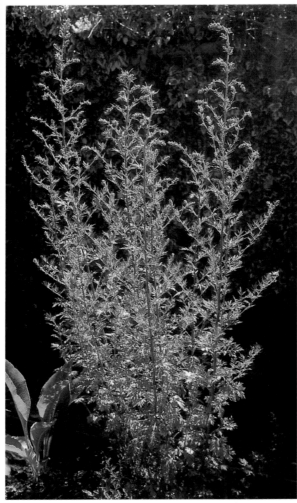

ARTEMISIA VULGARIS

Called the "mother of herbs," mugwort has been considered a magical herb in many cultures. It grows robustly along roadsides and is said to protect the traveler. In some traditions, it was hung in the house or made into amulets to keep away evil spirits. Mugwort also repels insects, including moths.

This is an herb with many actions. Best described as a tonic with particular application to the digestive and nervous systems, it reduces nervous indigestion, nausea and irritability. As a womb tonic it is useful to regulate periods, and reduce period pain and PMS. Fluff from the flowers is burnt as *moxa* in Chinese and Japanese medicine.

PARTS USED: Flowers and leaves.
DOSE: ¼ – ½ teaspoon three times a day.

CAUTION
Avoid during pregnancy.

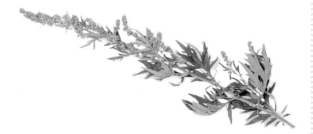

Mugwort is a sturdy tonic herb which can grow up to 3 feet high.

The gray-green foliage of mugwort shimmering at the roadside makes this a distinctive herb.

ST. JOHN'S WORT

HYPERICUM PERFORATUM

There are many plants in the St. John's wort family, but only the wild *Hypericum perforatum* has the tiny oil glands that contain hypericin. To be sure you have the right plant, hold up a leaf to the sun – the oil glands look like little holes, hence the name *perforatum*. The red oil stains your fingers when you pick the plant, and it is used externally to treat burns, neuralgia and inflammation. Some writers have associated this oil with the blood from St. John's beheading. An attractive pink infused oil can be made for external use. The plant thrives in the sunshine and springs up where trees have been felled.

Traditionally, St. John's wort was considered to be magically protective and a remedy for melancholy. It is now becoming well-known for its anti depressant action. It is a nerve tonic which helps both nervous exhaustion and damage to nerves caused by diseases such as shingles and herpes.

PARTS USED: The flowering tops.

DOSE: 1 teaspoon dried/2 teaspoons fresh to a cup of boiling water, three times a day.

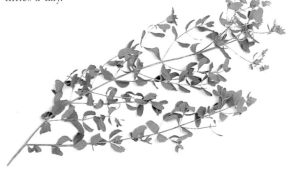

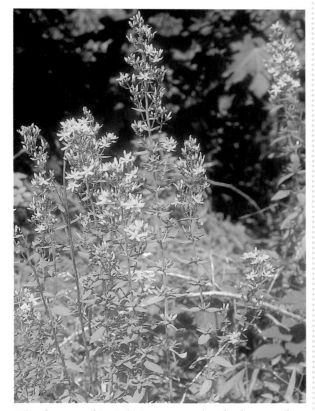

The flowers of St. John's wort need to be harvested as soon as they begin to open.

CAUTION
This remedy is best avoided when you are spending time in bright sunlight.

DAMIANA

TURNERA DIFFUSA

Damiana grows in South America and the West Indies. It was previously called *Turnera aphrodisiaca* and is a tonic to the nervous system and the reproductive system. It raises the spirits and is particularly useful if sexual function is impaired. It is traditionally a remedy for men, but the stimulant and tonic effects work well for women, too.

PARTS USED: Leaves and stem.

DOSE: 1 teaspoon to a cup of boiling water twice a day.

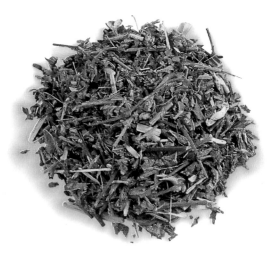

Damiana is harvested when flowering and dried for use as an antidepressant, to relieve anxiety and to improve sexual function.

WILD OATS

AVENA SATIVA

Oats are an excellent tonic to the nervous system, providing both nourishment and energy. Anybody who has seen the effects of oats on horses will understand their action. They are slightly stimulating and a long-term remedy for nervous exhaustion, lifting the mood while improving adaptability. Oats are also useful when there is disease of the nervous system such as shingles or herpes. A traditional breakfast of oatmeal is certainly a good idea. Oats contain vitamin E, iron, zinc, manganese and protein and are a good source of fiber, which helps to lower cholesterol levels.

PARTS USED: Seeds and stalks.

DOSE: There are many ways to eat oats – as oatmeal, pancakes, oatcakes and other dishes, as well as tea.

CAUTION
Oats are not suitable for those with a gluten sensitivity.

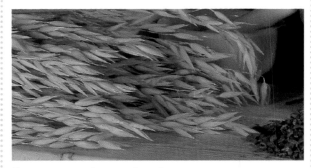

Oats are a good general tonic.

VERVAIN

VERBENA OFFICINALIS, HERB OF GRACE

An unassuming plant with tiny bluish-purple flowers that appears, like a mist, on waste ground and roadsides. Vervain has a long-documented reputation in the treatment of many physical and psychological problems. As a protective and purifying herb it was considered one of the most magical by both the Druids and the Romans – it has continued to be referred to in medical texts long after magic and medicine were separated.

Vervain is a nervous tonic with a slightly sedative action. It is useful for treating nervous exhaustion and symptoms of tension that include headaches and nausea. Vervain has also been used for gallbladder problems and depression and combines well with oats.

PARTS USED: Leaves and flowers.

DOSE: 1 teaspoon dried/2 teaspoons fresh to a cup of boiling water.

Lift your boughs of Vervain blue
Dipt in cold September dew
And dash the moisture chaste and clear,
O'er the ground and through the air.
Now the place is purged and pure.
WILLIAM MASON (1724 – 97)

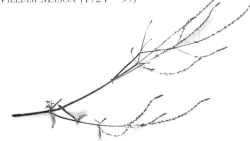

CRAMP BARK

VIBURNUM OPULUS, GUELDER ROSE

A decorative wild bush that produces glorious white and pale pink spring flowers, followed by red berries among its crimson foliage in autumn. Gardeners know it as the snowball bush. Geoffrey Grigson in *The Englishman's Flora* (1958) said it had a smell like crisply fried, well-peppered trout! The fruits have been used in preserves and as a substitute for cranberries, and a liquor has been distilled from them. They are very tart, but are good mixed with elder, rowan and blackberries in jam.

Therapeutically, the use of cramp bark is a good illustration of the connection between body and mind. It reduces spasm whatever the cause and is therefore helpful for constipation, period pains, high blood pressure and feeling "uptight."

PARTS USED: Dried bark.

DOSE: 1 teaspoon to a cup of boiling water.

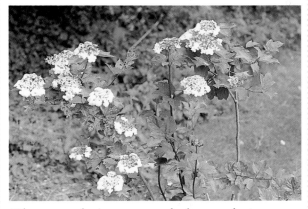

Viburnum opulus is a common hedgerow plant.

LAVENDER

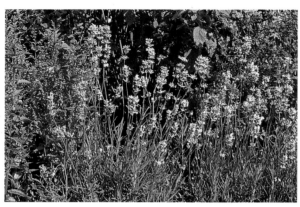

The lavender plant is always a delight.

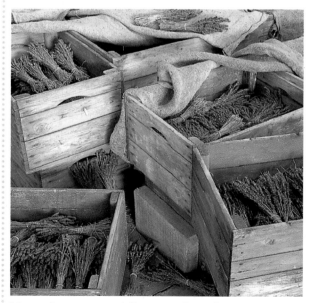

Harvesting commercially grown lavender.

LAVANDULA SPP.

Everybody knows this fragrant plant. Herbalists call it a thymoleptic, which means it raises the spirits. This, combined with its anti-infective action and relaxing properties, makes lavender a powerful remedy. The essential oil is used externally for relaxation and to heal sores and burns. It is less well-known that lavender can be taken internally in a tea or tincture. It reduces gas; indeed, lavender was at one time used as a condiment. The flowers can be used to flavor cookies, vinegar, desserts and ice creams. Lavender is an ideal remedy for irritation, indigestion and potential migraines. A few fresh or dried flowers added to teas made with other herbs, such as nettle, will have a cheering effect.

PARTS USED: Flowers and stalks.

DOSE: ½ teaspoon to a cup of boiling water 3 times a day. Use infused oil for massage or in the bath.

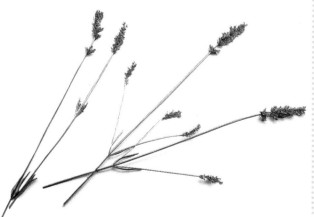

ROSEMARY

ROSMARINUS OFFICINALIS

A familiar plant containing several active, aromatic oils. This sturdy shrub is often found in gardens. Like lavender, it can be used both externally, in the form of essential or infused oil, and internally, as a flavoring, tea or tincture.

The actions of rosemary are centered on the head and womb. It increases the supply of blood to both. In the head it is helpful for cold headaches, forgetfulness (it symbolizes remembrance) and even premature baldness. In the womb and the gut it eases spasm due to poor circulation. With a general relaxing and anti-depressive action, this is a remedy appropriate for many problems associated with poor circulation.

Externally, the oil can be used as an antimicrobial remedy and to reduce pain as well as to clear the head.

PARTS USED: Leaves and flowers.

DOSE: 1 teaspoon to a cup of boiling water 3 times a day.

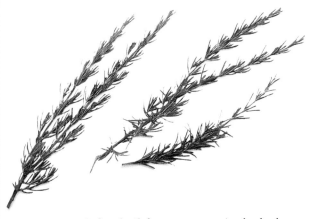

Use rosemary-infused oil for massage or in the bath.

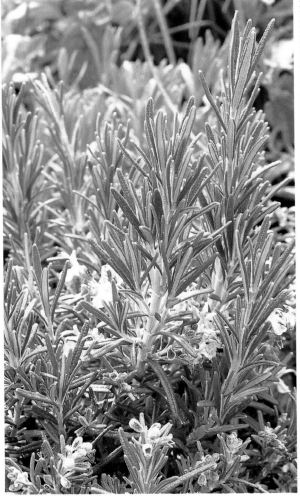

The Latin name for rosemary, *Rosmarinus officinalis*, means "dew of the sea."

MOTHERWORT

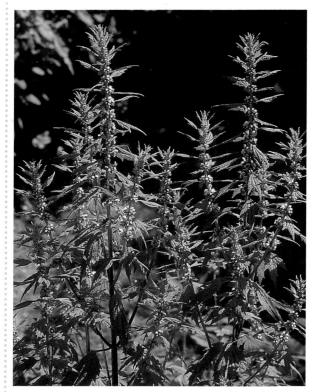

LEONURUS CARDIACA

This stately plant, with its strong, wine-colored square stem, bears delicate mauve flowers within prickly, toothed calyces. Its name is thought to refer to the leaves being the shape of a lion's tail, and *cardiaca* implies that this herb will strengthen the heart. In Britain it used to be grown for use as a remedy, while in the rest of Europe it is found wild. Motherwort makes a fine syrup and a refreshing, bitter tea.

It is a great calmer, especially if tension is causing palpitations or sweats. It improves and tones the circulatory system and is useful for relieving menstrual and menopausal problems. Motherwort can help lower blood pressure and improve cardiac output during exercise.

According to Culpeper, it makes mothers joyful. It combines well with lady's mantle.

PARTS USED: Leaves and flowers.

DOSE: 1 teaspoon dried/2 teaspoons fresh to a cup of boiling water 3 times a day, or 2 teaspoons syrup.

Motherwort requires moist soil and good drainage.

CAUTION
Avoid during the first trimester of pregnancy.

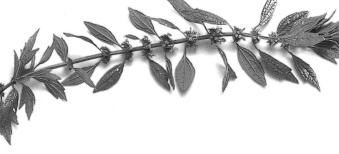

Motherwort has always been associated with the sun.

CHASTE TREE

VITEX AGNUS-CASTUS, MONK'S PEPPER

The berries from this aromatic wayside bush found in southern Europe have a tradition of use by both women and men. Its common name reflects a slight anti-estrogen effect which can cool passion; perhaps this property may account for its other common name – Monk's Pepper.

Many menstrual problems are a result of an excess of estrogen, possibly due to use of the contraceptive pill or environmental pollution. Small doses of chaste tree can re-balance the hormones and reduce some of the symptoms of PMS, menopausal change, infertility, postnatal depression and irregular periods. It also increases milk production after birth. Altogether it is a soothing and much appreciated plant.

PARTS USED: Dried ripe fruits.

DOSE: 10 – 20 drops of tincture taken first thing in the morning.

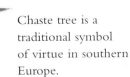

Chaste tree is a traditional symbol of virtue in southern Europe.

LADY'S MANTLE

ALCHEMILLA XANTHOCHLORA syn.
A. VULGARIS, VIRGIN'S CAPE

The unusual leaves of this plant resemble a cloak – hence its common names. Each leaf collects a shining drop of dew overnight. The name *Alchemilla* derives from the Arabic word for alchemy, a reference to its power to make a change. A larger species, *Alchemilla mollis,* is often grown as a foliage plant in gardens – it is thought to have similar properties.

As its name suggests, lady's mantle is a woman's herb; like chaste tree, it helps balance menstrual cycles. As a douche or wash, an infusion soothes itching and inflammation. A warming, drying remedy, it is useful for excessive bleeding and diarrhea.

PARTS USED: Leaves and flowers.

DOSE: 1 teaspoon dried/2 teaspoons fresh to a cup of boiling water 3 times a day.

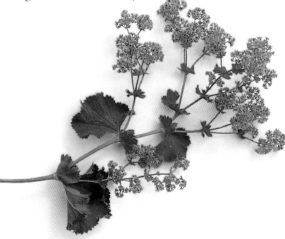

Alchemilla mollis.

EVENING PRIMROSE

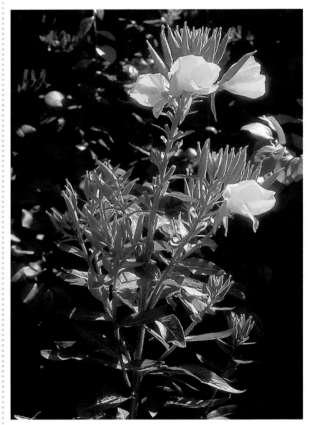

OENOTHERA BIENNIS

A beautiful plant, luminous in the twilight, evening primrose is generous in its actions and appearance. A statuesque plant growing over 3 feet tall, its large, pale, yellow flowers open in the early evening and quickly fade to be replaced by tubular seed pods. It produces many seeds and spreads freely.

The whole plant is edible; the oil from the seeds is a source of essential fatty acids and is therefore useful as a nutritional supplement. It is also used externally for eczema and other dry skin conditions. Taken internally, evening primrose oil reduces cholesterol levels and benefits the circulation generally. Supplements are recommended for sufferers from rheumatoid arthritis, multiple sclerosis and diabetes. Evening primrose oil can also be helpful for PMS and other inflammatory conditions.

PARTS USED: Oil produced from seeds.
DOSE: Capsules as directed.

CAUTION
Avoid in cases of epilepsy.

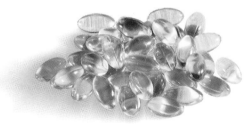

Above: The evening primrose likes to grow in dry, sunny conditions. Although the flowers of *Oenothera* each last only a short time, they are produced in succession.

Right: Evening primrose capsules are readily available commercially.

LIME BLOSSOM

TILIA x EUROPAEA, LINDEN BLOSSOM

Found, according to Culpeper, "in parks and gentle-men's gardens," the tall, upstanding lime tree with its warm, honey-scented blossom is a real favorite. Lime blossom honey is prized and the infusion *tilleul* is popular in France. Grigson warned you should pick your own flowers because those harvested and dried commercially taste of newspaper!

The pale, soft wood of lime trees is used for delicate carving and produces artist's charcoal. The fibers are used in basketry and rope-making.

Lime is no less useful medicinally, being relaxing and cleansing. It makes a helpful tea for fevers and flu, especially if combined with yarrow and peppermint. It encourages sweating and thus helps the body through fevers. It is also used to reduce hardening of the arteries and high blood pressure. It can relieve vascular headaches, including migraine.

Lime blossom combines well with lemon balm to ease nervous tension.

PARTS USED: Flowers, including the pale, yellowish bracts.

DOSE: 1 teaspoon dried/2 teaspoons fresh to a cup of boiling water 3 times a day.

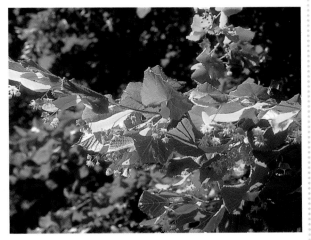

The deliciously scented flowers of the lime tree should be collected when they have just opened.

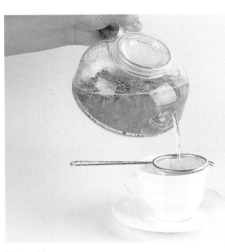

Lime blossom tea.

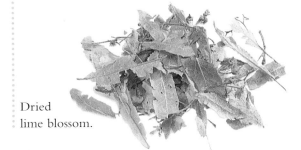

Dried lime blossom.

41

MINT

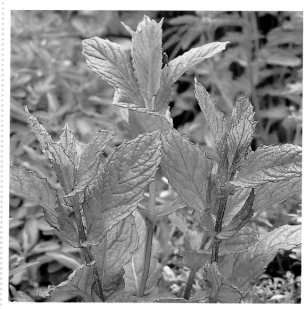

Peppermint has to be propagated by root division in the spring. It is an invasive plant and needs cutting back regularly.

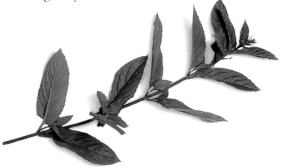

MENTHA SPP.

Peppermint (*Mentha piperita*) is the most used of the mint family, and is a hybrid between spearmint and watermint, but most mints have some therapeutic effect. The plants are robust and spread enthusiastically, although they need plenty of moisture to grow well. Peppermint seems always to have been popular; there is evidence that it was cultivated by the Egyptians and certainly the Greeks and Romans used it. Roman women ate it after drinking wine to mask the breath.

Mint is used as flavoring and medicine, chiefly because of the action of volatile oils. This is a cheerful plant that reduces spasm in the gut and increases the production of digestive secretions. It's easy to see why after-dinner mints are so popular. Mint is also used in drinks, jellies and sauces.

Peppermint is antiseptic and anti-parasitic, and will reduce itching. It has a temporary anesthetic effect on the skin and gives the impression of cooling. It is included in lotions for massaging aching muscles, and makes an effective footbath for tired, hot feet.

It is included in traditional teas for alleviating the symptoms of colds and flu.

PARTS USED: Leaves and flowers.

DOSE: 1 teaspoon dried/2 teaspoons fresh to a cup of boiling water.

CAUTION
Excessive use of mint can damage the gut or cause headaches. Avoid it if you have a peptic ulcer.

PASQUE FLOWER

ANEMONE PULSATILLA, WIND FLOWER

This is perhaps one of the most beautiful medicinal herbs. The vivid, purple flowers appear among grayish foliage in the spring and are therefore named for Easter (from the Middle English word *Pasch*).

Pasque Flower is a sedative, bactericidal, anti-spasmodic painkiller, with a particular affinity with the reproductive organs. Thus, it is used for all types of pain affecting male and female genital organs, with or without an element of tension or agitation.

PARTS USED: Dried leaves and flowers.

DOSE: A very low dose is needed – it is advisable to consult an herbalist or buy a commercial preparation.

CAUTION
Do not use the fresh plant.

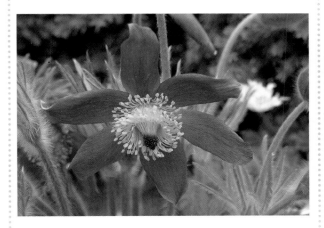

The delicate Pasque flower is now a rarity in the wild.

MARJORAM

ORIGANUM VULGARE

There are many species of marjoram, whose botanical name comes from the Greek and means "joy of the mountain." Sweet marjoram (*Origanum majorana*) is commonly used in potpourri, and as a culinary herb it is popular in Greek and Italian cooking. Wild marjoram, usually referred to as oregano when used in cooking, has a spicy fragrance, small, rounded leaves and tiny, pink flowers.

Medicinally, marjoram reduces depression and is helpful for nervous headaches. It contains volatile oils that are antispasmodic so it is useful in soothing digestive upsets.

The infused oil can be used in the bath to relieve stiffness or rubbed onto sore and aching joints or muscles.

PARTS USED: Leaves.

DOSE: 1 teaspoon dried/2 teaspoons fresh to a cup of boiling water, twice a day.

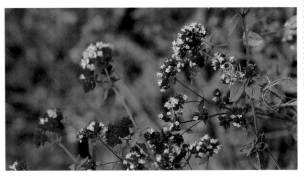

The oil distilled from marjoram is used commercially in toiletries and perfumes.

HERBAL RECIPES

YOU CAN'T ALWAYS AVOID STRESS, but there are plenty of things you can do to help yourself cope better when life presents a challenge.

Diet really does make a difference. Make sure you eat proper, healthy meals with lots of vitamin-rich fruits and vegetables and no artificial additives (add herbs instead, to contribute flavor to your food as well as extra goodness).

Try to reduce stimulants such as tea, coffee, alcohol and cola – drink plenty of water or herbal tea. Exercise is important too; it dispels excess adrenaline and improves relaxation and sleep.

Stressful events are likely to disrupt your appetite and your ability to rest, but both are vital to enable you to cope well. Use herbal remedies as your allies to improve your digestion, help you relax and improve your adaptability.

The recipes that follow are designed to help

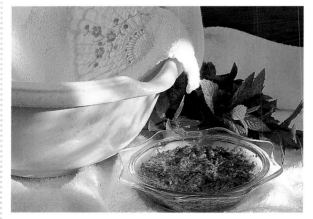

Peppermint is cooling and counteracts tiredness. The essential oil is ideal for using in a refreshing footbath.

you through some of the difficult periods that assail everyone from time to time. As long as you don't exceed the doses stated, and as long as you are sure you are using the right plant, it is safe to experiment with these suggestions to find the best remedy for you. But remember to seek professional help if a problem persists.

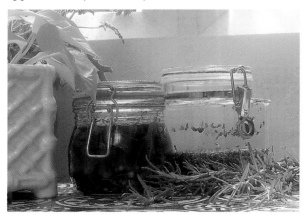

Herbs in many forms: lavender as an infused oil, lime blossom as a tincture and fresh rosemary stems.

Facing page: Handling herbs and preparing herbal teas and other recipes can be a relaxing experience.

44

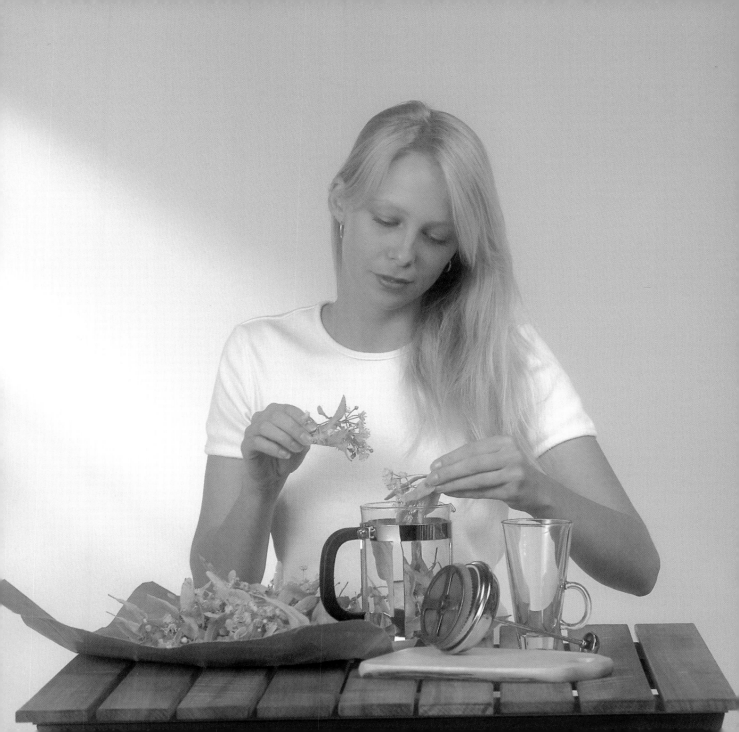

PREPARING FOR A BIG DAY

If you are getting ready for an important event in your life, you are bound to want to be sure that you will cope well. If you are preparing for exams or some other important test, you'll need to be able to concentrate when you are working, but also be able to switch off and rest when you stop.

As well as paying special attention to your diet, you might take a multivitamin supplement or yeast tablets to nourish your nervous system with plenty of vitamin B. Try to get regular exercise, and release the build-up of tension with a relaxing massage or even just an herbal bath. However busy you are, try to do something for pleasure each day.

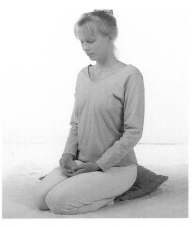

Use meditation to calm the mind and help you wind down.

SUSTAINING TEA

Boil 1 teaspoon each dried licorice and ginseng root in 2½ cups water for 10 minutes. Pour the decoction over 3 teaspoons dried borage. Let steep for 10 minutes. Strain.

Drink one cupful, hot or cold, three times a day.

OTHER SUGGESTIONS

• Make borage tea and sweeten to taste with a solid bar of licorice.
• Buy ginseng capsules and take as directed for three weeks before the big event.
• Eat a big bowl of oatmeal for breakfast every morning.
• Treat yourself to a pancake.

CAUTION
Licorice is not recommended for those with high blood pressure.

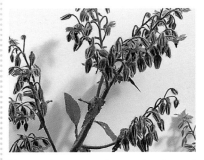

Borage improves the production of adrenaline in times of stress.

HERBAL REMEDIES THAT WILL HELP
• Ginseng (*Panax* for men and *Eleutherococcus* for women)
• Wild oats
• Licorice
• Borage

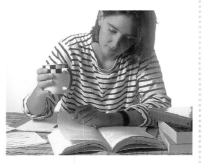

Ginseng helps concentration and improves clarity of mind.

COPING WITH A DIFFICULT TIME

However well you normally manage, sometimes life just gets hard. Maybe there's a new baby in the family, a relative is ill and depending on you, you're moving or you're very busy at work. It's important to remember to take care of yourself when extra demands are made on you. Diet, sleep and exercise are all crucial, and herbs can help during stressful times.

HERBAL REMEDIES THAT WILL HELP
- Wild oats
- Licorice
- Borage
- Skullcap, wood betony or vervain, according to your usual reaction to stress

DE-STRESSING TEA
Put 1 teaspoon of each of the dried herbs listed above into a pitcher, teapot or cafetière. Add boiling water and let infuse for 10 minutes. Strain and sweeten with more licorice (avoid if you have high blood pressure). Drink one cup, warm, three times a day.

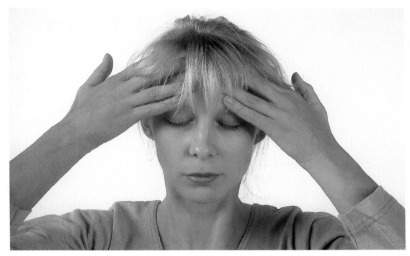

Rub a little lavender oil on the temples and forehead when you are under pressure to help you relax.

Skullcap calms anxiety.

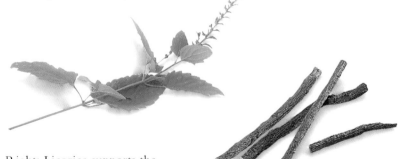

Right: Licorice supports the adrenal glands.

RELIEVING PMS

Women experience a variety of symptoms before their period. Sometimes it can be good to acknowledge that you are cyclic and changeable and need, if you can, to do different things at different times in the month. Unfortunately, this isn't always possible. If you feel too much "not yourself" at this time, it may help you to eat particularly vitamin- and mineral-rich foods. For the second half of your cycle, eat plenty of fruit and salad, especially bananas, carrots, nuts and grapes. Cut right down on salt and processed food, and eat little and often to avoid cravings.

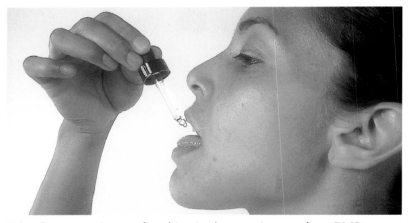

Take chaste tree tincture first thing in the morning to relieve PMS.

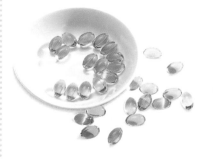

Capsules of evening primrose oil provide essential fatty acids, often lacking with PMS.

HERBAL REMEDIES
THAT WILL HELP
• Chaste tree
• Evening primrose
• Vervain
• Lady's mantle

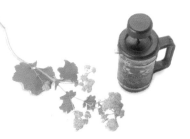

A LONG-TERM SOLUTION

Take chaste tree tincture, 12 drops every morning for three months. Take evening primrose oil capsules as directed on the packet.

VERVAIN AND LADY'S MANTLE TEA

Put 1 teaspoon each dried vervain and dried lady's mantle into a pot. Add 1¼ cups boiling water. Steep for 10 minutes. Strain and sweeten to taste.

Take one cup twice a day from day 14 of your cycle, or two weeks after your period starts.

EASING PERIOD PAIN

Pain during or just before periods is due to contractions in the muscles of the womb that reduce blood flow, causing the muscles to ache. Exercise and heat will increase the circulation of blood.

Cramp bark, as its name implies, reduces spasm, and rosemary is a circulatory stimulant, particularly associated with the womb and the head. Its aromatic oils are uplifting and relaxing. A decoction of ginger, drunk frequently before and during your period, is helpful too.

A hot water bottle can be comforting, but for added benefit try using a hot, aromatic compress.

HERBAL REMEDIES THAT WILL HELP
- Cramp bark
- Rosemary
- Ginger

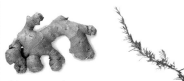

Ginger and rosemary.

CRAMP BARK AND ROSEMARY COMPRESS

1 Boil 2 teaspoons cramp bark in 2½ cups water for 10 to 15 minutes. Add 2 teaspoons dried rosemary. Let steep for 15 minutes, then strain.

2 Soak a clean cotton cloth or bandage in the liquid. When cool enough to handle, wring out the cloth.

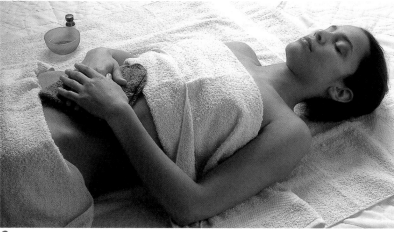

3 Place the hot compress on your abdomen and relax.

HELPING WITH MENOPAUSE

Menopause doesn't have to be a problem, but the changes in women's lives and bodies can cause difficulties. Think of these years as a time to look after yourself and rethink old habits.

HERBAL REMEDIES THAT WILL HELP
- Chaste tree
- Motherwort
- Sage
- Lime blossom
- Licorice

WHEN YOUR PERIODS FIRST BECOME IRREGULAR
Take 10 drops of chaste tree tincture each morning for three months.

REDUCING NIGHT SWEATS
Dissolve 1 teaspoon honey in a cup of hot water. Add 2 drops of sage essential oil.

Drink the mixture before you go to bed, then cover yourself with a dry towel and rest. Add any remaining tea to your bath water the following day.

ALLEVIATING HOT SWEATS

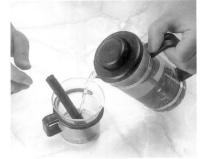

1 Put 1 teaspoon each dried motherwort and sage in a cup. Pour on 2½ cups boiling water. Sweeten with licorice (omit this if you have high blood pressure).

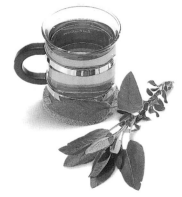

2 Let cool, then sip throughout the day.

CAUTION
Do not drink sage tea continually. Take for three weeks, then avoid for at least one week.

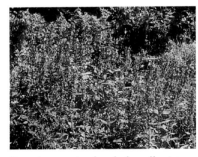

Sage is a tonic that helps alleviate stress due to change.

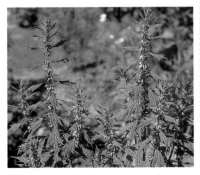

Motherwort helps to strengthen the heart.

RELAXING TENSE MUSCLES

Muscles can become tense as a result of anxiety; this often causes slightly raised shoulders or contracted back muscles. The effort of maintaining your muscles in this semi-contracted state is tiring and may eventually result in perpetual spasm and bad postural habits. Your neck will feel stiff and your back may ache. Tight neck muscles can also prevent adequate blood flow to your head and cause tension headaches.

Another cause of muscle tension is spending a long time in the same position. This can occur if you are bending your head to look at a computer screen or driving a long distance. It's important to move frequently to release the muscles. Rotate your head or stand up and stretch, and remember to take regular breaks from

HERBAL REMEDIES THAT WILL HELP
- Lavender
- Marjoram
- Rosemary
- Cramp bark

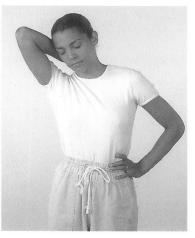

Tension can build up in the neck and shoulders, causing stiffness.

working or driving. Massaging the neck and shoulders with a relaxing oil can help.

COLD INFUSED OIL OF LAVENDER
Fill a jar with lavender heads and cover with clear vegetable oil. Let steep on a windowsill for a month, shaking the jar every day. Strain and bottle.

Massage into a stiff neck or back. This oil can also be added to the bath to keep your skin soft and perfumed while encouraging

relaxation. Similar oils can be made from marjoram (which is antispasmodic) or rosemary.

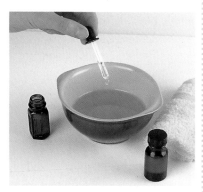

Dilute concentrated essential oil before use on the skin. Add 2 drops of oil to 4 teaspoons of grapeseed or almond oil.

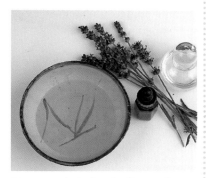

Homemade infused oils are cheap to make and very effective.

CALMING ANXIETY

We all know what it feels like to be excited – just remember waiting for a party when you were a child. This is a great part of life, but inappropriate or excessive excitement, often combined with frustration, will lead to anxiety. Think of a commuter pacing up and down the station platform, late for a meeting, or a parent tossing and turning in bed when their teenage child is still out late at night. In situations like these you are producing too much adrenaline. Your body is primed for "fight or flight" with nowhere to go. Your heart is racing, your muscles are tense and your chest is expanded. All these conditions are appropriate before a race, but not in bed or on the train.

Anxiety can cause many symptoms, including palpitations, sweating, irritability and sleeplessness. Herbs can help very effectively with all of these.

Rescue Remedy, a Bach Flower Remedy readily available over the counter, can be used if you feel frightened or anxious – just put two drops on your tongue.

HERBAL REMEDIES
THAT WILL HELP
- *To help your nervous system adapt:*
  - Wild oats
  - Vervain
  - St. John's wort
  - Skullcap
  - Wood betony

These are all nervous tonics. Choose whichever one suits you best and combine it with a specific remedy for the symptom that troubles you most.
- *To ease palpitations:* Motherwort or Passionflower
- *To reduce sweating:* Valerian or Motherwort
- *To help you sleep:* Passionflower or Valerian

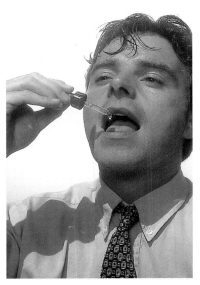

Two drops of Rescue Remedy on the tongue can help prevent a panic attack.

Motherwort relieves palpitations.

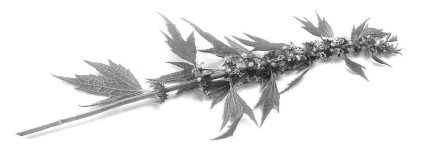

Long-term Treatment for Anxiety

Put 1 teaspoon of each of your three chosen dried herbs into a pot (use only ½ teaspoon Passionflower). Add 2½ cups boiling water and let steep for 10 – 15 minutes. Strain.

Sit down and drink one cup three times a day. Do this for at least two to four weeks.

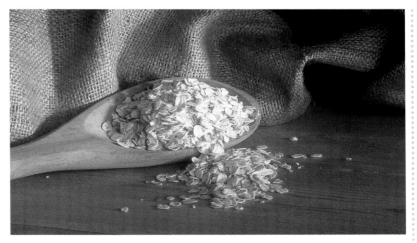

Above: Oats are a food for both the body and the mind.

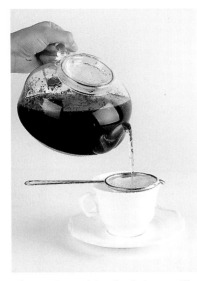

Above: A soothing herbal tea will help to reduce overreaction.

Right: Lavender and hops both reduce tension and encourage relaxing sleep.

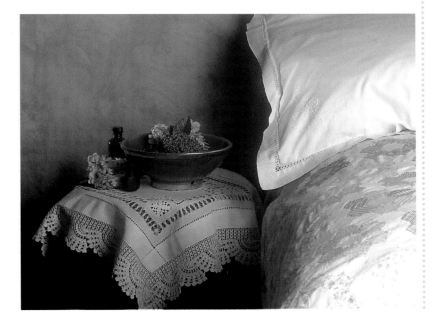

RECOVERING FROM NERVOUS EXHAUSTION

You are much more likely to get ill or depressed after or during a long period of hard work or heavy emotional demands. This can easily happen to teachers at the end of term, or to those who care for disabled or sick relatives on a long-term basis. Herbal remedies will give your nervous system some support at times like this.

HERBAL REMEDIES THAT WILL HELP
- Wild oats
- Licorice
- St. John's wort
- Skullcap
- Borage
- Wood betony

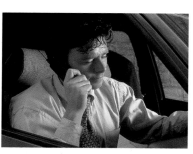

Try to find ways to reduce the impact of everyday stress.

REVITALIZING TEA
Mix equal portions of all the dried herbs listed. Put 4 teaspoons of the mixture into a pot with a lid. Add 2½ cups boiling water. Let steep for 10 minutes. Strain.

Drink three or four cups of this tea a day.

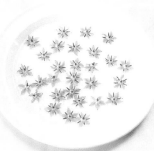

The delicate, star-shaped flowers of borage help to raise the spirits.

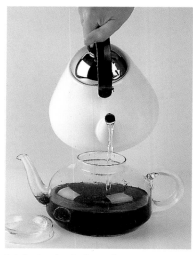

Make an herbal tea from a blend of supportive herbs when you are feeling exhausted.

Wood betony.

54

TONICS FOR CONVALESCENCE

It is easy to forget that, even if your symptoms have gone, your body needs time to recover after an illness. Dealing with disease depletes your immune system and, if you do not give yourself time to recoup, you will become more vulnerable to post-viral syndrome or recurrent infections. The old-fashioned concept of a tonic is useful. Wild oats and St. John's wort support the nervous system, vervain promotes relaxation and digestion and licorice and borage restore the adrenal glands.

Vitamin C supplements should be continued for several weeks after an illness – take at least 1–2 grams each day. Plenty of rest is important, as is a nourishing diet. Alfalfa sprouts are a rich source of vitamins and minerals.

TONIC TEA
Put ½ teaspoon of each of the listed dried herbs into a small pot. Add boiling water. Flavor with peppermint or licorice to taste.

(Avoid licorice if you suffer from high blood pressure.) Let steep for 10 minutes. Strain. Drink three or four cups, warm, each day for at least three weeks.

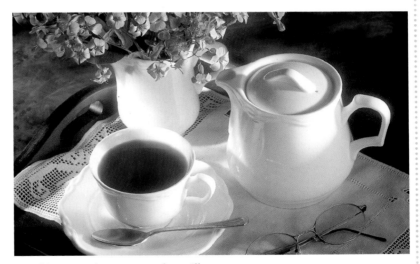

Drinking a tonic tea every day will encourage recovery.

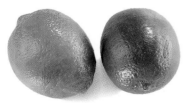

Citrus fruits are a well-known source of vitamin C.

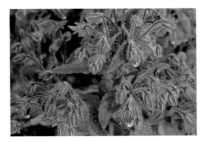

Borage restores the adrenal glands.

HERBAL REMEDIES THAT WILL HELP
- Wild oats
- Vervain
- St. John's wort
- Borage
- Licorice

RELIEVING WINTER BLUES

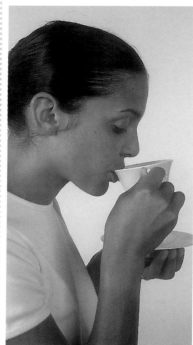

Try some of the many different herb teas to find one you enjoy.

HERBAL REMEDIES THAT WILL HELP
- St. John's wort
- Wild oats
- Ginseng
- Rosemary

The old herbalists thought that the appearance of a plant held a clue to its healing action. For instance, pilewort (lesser celandine) has roots that resemble hemorrhoids, and it does indeed make an effective ointment for piles. The flowers of St. John's wort resemble nothing so much as the sun. The plant thrives in sunlight and is known to have antidepressant effects. There is no better herb than this to take if you are depressed in the winter, when sunlight is in short supply.

Wild oats also help by strengthening the nervous system and keeping you warm. Rosemary, an evergreen plant, will improve circulation to the head and keep the mind clear.

Ginseng capsules can be taken for a month in the early autumn to help you adapt to the transition between seasons.

WINTER BRIGHTENER
Combine 2 teaspoons dried St. John's wort with 1 teaspoon dried rosemary. Add 1 cup boiling water. Let steep for 10 minutes. Strain.
Drink three times a day throughout the winter.

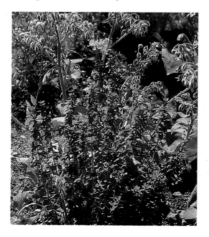

St. John's wort thrives in sunlight.

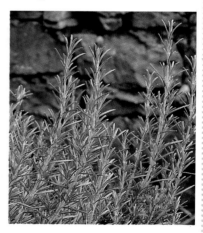

Rosemary helps to clear the mind.

LIFTING DEPRESSION

Depression illustrates the connection between body and mind. Physical and emotional energy are both depleted when you are in a depressed state. Both will benefit from a healthy diet with plenty of raw, vital foods, nuts, seeds and vitamin B. A multivitamin and mineral supplement may be useful until you feel energetic enough to prepare good food. Try also to cut down on stimulants, such as caffeine, that tend to depress both body and mind.

The restorative tea suggested will restore the health of your nervous system while having a slightly stimulating effect.

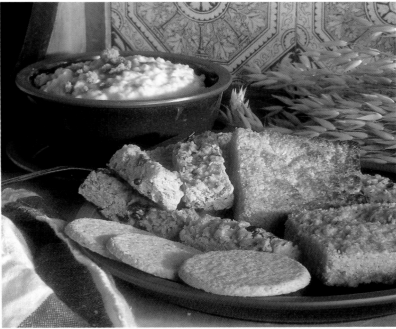

There are many tasty ways to include the goodness of oats in your diet.

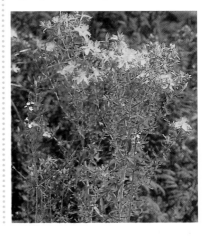

St. John's wort is a nerve tonic.

HERBAL REMEDIES THAT WILL HELP
- St. John's wort
- Wild oats
- Damiana

RESTORATIVE TEA

Mix equal parts of each of the dried herbs listed. Put 2 teaspoons of the mixture into a pot. Add 2½ cups boiling water. Let steep for 10 minutes and then strain.

Drink one cup of this tea three times a day.

DIGESTIVES

Many people suffer from digestive upsets when they are stressed. This is because the "fight-or-flight" activity of the sympathetic nervous system tends to suppress digestive processes. The result may be indigestion, loss of appetite, wind, diarrhea or irritable bowel.

The recipes below will relax the nervous system, encouraging parasympathetic activity and reducing spasm in the gut.

HERBAL REMEDIES THAT WILL HELP
- Chamomile
- Lemon balm
- Peppermint
- Licorice
- Cramp bark
- Hops
- Fennel, caraway, dill, cumin

TO CALM BUTTERFLIES, OR A NERVOUS STOMACH
Chamomile, hops and lemon balm can be combined in a tea, or select the best combination for

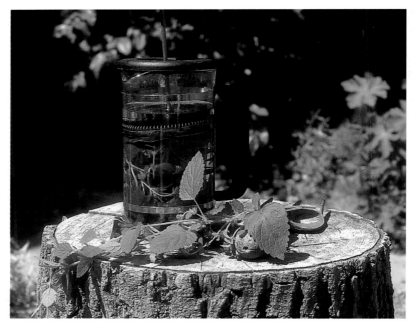

you. Lemon balm and chamomile can be taken as frequently as you find suitable.

Put 1 teaspoon each lemon balm, dried chamomile flowers and peppermint into a small teapot or cafetière. Add a mug of boiling water and let steep for at least 10 minutes. Strain and drink at least three times a day or after meals. Hops can be added to settle the stomach in the evening.

Fresh lemon balm makes a delicious tea and calms the stomach.

CAUTION
Hops are a sedative, so should only be added at night. Avoid hops if you are depressed or lacking in sexual energy. Avoid licorice if you have high blood pressure.

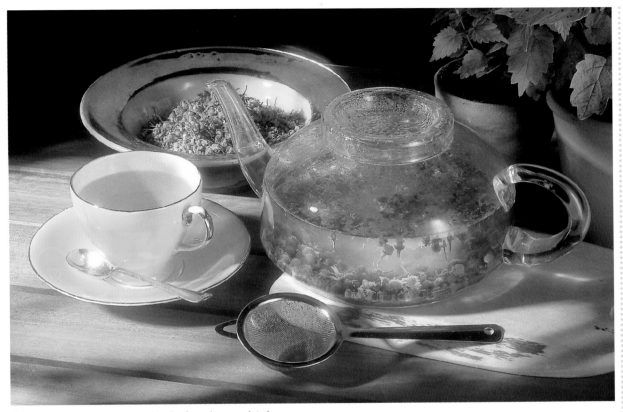

Chamomile tea makes an ideal after-dinner drink.

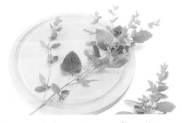

Lemon balm acts as a digestive.

TO RELIEVE WIND AND COLIC

Boil 1 teaspoon each fennel seeds and cramp bark in about 1¼ cups water. Add 1 teaspoon dried peppermint. Let steep for 10 minutes. Strain and drink.

TO EASE CONSTIPATION

Make a decoction of cramp bark and fennel as above, but add 1 teaspoon licorice root.

If constipation is a recurrent condition, 1 teaspoon linseeds added to your breakfast cereal can be helpful in relieving it.

HANGOVER REMEDIES

Most people know what a hangover feels like – a combination of headache, nausea, fuzzy head and depression. Most of these symptoms are connected with the liver being overloaded and unable to perform its many crucial functions properly. Bitter herbs stimulate the liver and hurry along its detoxification work. Vervain is bitter and lavender aids digestion; both herbs lift the spirits.

If you have a hangover, it is also advisable to drink plenty of water and take extra vitamin C.

HERBAL REMEDIES THAT WILL HELP
- Vervain
- Lavender

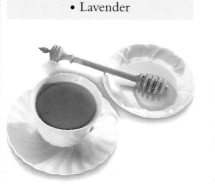

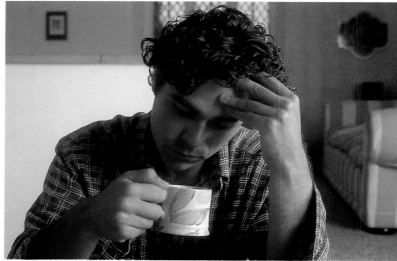

Herbal comfort for the morning after.

MORNING-AFTER TEA

Put 1 teaspoon dried vervain and ½ teaspoon lavender flowers into a pot. Add 2½ cups boiling water and cover to keep in the volatile oils. Let steep for 10 minutes. Strain and sweeten with a little honey.

Sip this tea as often as you like throughout the day until you start to feel better.

Add honey to sweeten any tea or decoction.

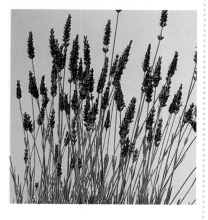

The lavender plant even looks calming.

RELIEVING TENSION HEADACHES

Headaches are a common symptom of stress. Often they are caused by tension in the neck and upper back muscles. This can prevent adequate blood supply to the head and thus lead to pain. Both massage and exercise can be a great help in easing this kind of headache.

HERBAL REMEDIES THAT WILL HELP
- Lavender
- Rosemary
- Wood betony

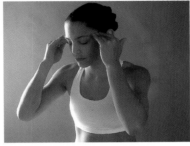

Lavender or rosemary oil can be rubbed into the temples.

SOOTHING TEA
Put 1 teaspoon dried wood betony and ½ teaspoon dried lavender or rosemary into a cup. Add boiling water and let steep for 10 minutes.

Strain and drink. Repeat hourly throughout the day.

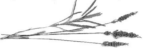

LAVENDER OR ROSEMARY SCENTED BATH
Pour a few drops of essential oil or some infused oil into a hot bath. Lie back and relax! Even better, tie a bunch of the fresh herb under the hot tap as you fill the bath (this avoids oily smears around the bath).

Two drops of essential oil of lavender can be mixed with 1 teaspoon hot or cold water and rubbed directly onto the head during times of stress.

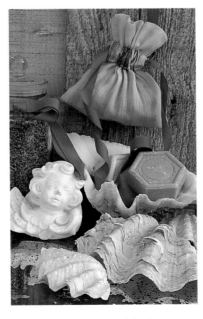

Hang a muslin bag of fresh or dried herbs under the hot tap.

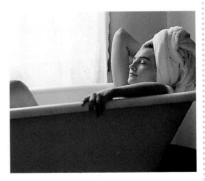

Make time to relax completely in a hot, scented bath.

Essential oil of rosemary.

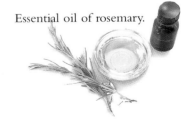

REVITALIZING THE LIBIDO

Sometimes depression or anxiety makes happy sexual functioning difficult. This may be because your energy is too low, or it may be connected with a hormone imbalance. Damiana stimulates both the nervous and hormonal systems. It has constituents which convert in the body to hormones. Vervain releases tension and stress and was traditionally used as an aphrodisiac. Wild oats and ginger are both stimulating too.

HERBAL REMEDIES THAT WILL HELP
- Damiana
- Vervain
- Wild oats
- Ginger

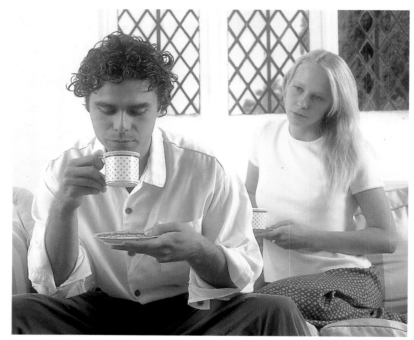

Herbs can help restore energy of all kinds, including sexual energy.

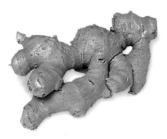

Ginger fires the blood.

ENERGIZING TEA
Put 1 teaspoon dried damiana and 1 teaspoon dried vervain into a pot. Add 2½ cups of boiling water. Let steep for 10 minutes.

Strain and flavor with licorice, ginger or honey. Drink two cups a day.

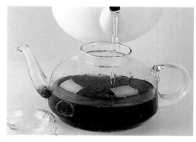

Dried herb tea.

ENHANCING SLEEP

There are many types of insomnia and many types of people. If you can't sleep it is best to experiment with the remedies below to find the one herb or combination of herbs which suits you. If you haven't been sleeping well for a long period, include a nervous system tonic to improve the long-term situation.

Drink teas made from relaxing herbs in the evenings. Lavender oil in a hot bath before bed and on the pillow will help. You could try a hop pillow, too.

Remember to allow time at the end of the day to relax and wind down. Exercise, meditation and yoga all help with sleep difficulties.

SLEEPY TEA
Put 1 teaspoon each dried chamomile, vervain and lemon balm into a pot. Add about 2½ cups boiling water. Let steep for 10 minutes.

Strain and drink one cup after supper. Warm the rest and drink before going to bed.

If you continue to have problems sleeping, add a decoction of 1 teaspoon valerian root or ½ teaspoon dried hops or Californian poppy to the herb blend.

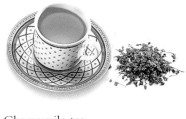

Chamomile tea.

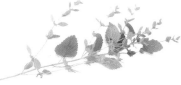

Lemon balm.

HERBAL REMEDIES THAT WILL HELP
- Lemon balm
- Chamomile
- Valerian
- Californian poppy
- Vervain
- Passionflower (use only ½ teaspoon a day)
- Hops (use ½ teaspoon a day)

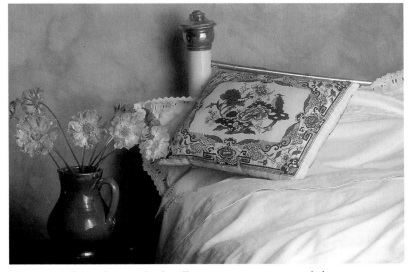

You can make or buy an herb pillow to encourage sound sleep.

INDEX AND ACKNOWLEDGMENTS

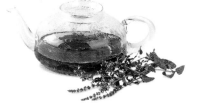

Acknowledgments:
The majority of photographs in this
book were taken by Don Last. The
pictures on pages 30l, 43bl were lent
by A-Z Botanical. The publishers
would also like to thank the following photographers for their contri-
butions: Polly Wreford, pages 23l,
37r, 42t; Debbie Patterson, pages 7tr,
21, 36bl; Lucy Mason, pages 6, 12l,
13tr, 14bl, 22bl, 28b, 29r, 34l, 36t,
39r, 41br, 46bl, 49bl, 51tr, 51br, 53l,
54tr, 56br, 60br; John Freeman and
Michelle Garrett, pages 9tl, 26t, 27t,
28t, 29l, 32br, 33bl, 39l, 43r;
Michelle Garrett, pages 10t, 44r,
61bl; Alistair Hughes, page 61ml;
and Sue Hawkey, page 35r.
t=top, b=bottom, r=right, l=left,
m=middle. The publishers would
also like to thank Andrew Tregear of
The Plantation, Harington Place,
Bath, for kindly providing baskets.

Author's Acknowledgments:
Thanks to my colleagues and
teachers from the National Institute
of Medical Herbalists and The
School of Phytotherapy, and to my
editor Fiona Eaton, who was fun to
work with.

Bibliography:
Grieve, Maud, *A Modern Herbal*,
  Jonathan Cape 1931, revised 1992
Grigson, Geoffrey, *The Englishman's
  Flora*, Phoenix House 1938